How to get Abs

# Contents

# want this?

30 jumping jacks
5 pushups
25 high knees
10 crunches
7 squats
30 butt kicks
5 pushups
10 crunches
30 jumping jacks
1 minute wall sit
10 crunches
repeat 2x

# you're one step closer

Flat stomach exercises

Who doesn't want that very flattering flat abs. Get into shape easy and fast with these easy and simple exercises. Also get firmer thighs and back while you are at it!

## Pike and Extend

Lie down on the floor. Facing upwards, extend your legs over hips with arms extended overhead. Now crunch up trying to reach your feet.

Now keeping your legs straight, bring your arms overhead while lowering upper back and left leg towards the floor. Again crunch up, raising your left leg over your hips while trying to touch your toes. Repeat the same with opposite legs.

## Side crunch while standing

Stand on left leg with left arm extended outwards at the height of the shoulder. Right foot should be lifted a few inches above the floor to the side. Place right hand behind your head with elbows bent out side wards at shoulder level. Then raise your right knee towards right elbow. Switch sides and repeat.

## Chest fly with extended legs

Lie on the floor while facing upwards. Knees need to bend at 90 degrees over hips. Hold a dumbbell in each hand while your arms are extended over your chest while palms facing in wards. Keep right knee bent while straightening left leg toward the floor as you lower your arms towards the sides. Hold for a while and return to top. Switch legs and repeat.

## Knee up with overhead press

Sit on the floor while bending your knees and feet firmly on the floor. Hold your dumbbells near the shoulder with elbows by your side and palms facing inwards. Lean backwards and stretch your arms overhead as you lift your feet a few inches above the floor while brining your knees towards the chest. Hold position and count to 3. Repeat about 15 times for best results.

## Lunge and twist

Stand upright with feet together. Lunge backwards with your left leg while bending your knees at 90 degrees. Try to reach your right foot with your left hand. Stand up again and raise your left knee in front to the height of your hip. Bring your fists closer to your chest while bending elbows out to your sides as you twist to your left. Then twist back to centre and lunge left leg back. Repeat the whole process and switch sides.

## Clock exercise

Using an exercise ball, rest your back on it while your feet is aligned with your hips. Stretch arms over your head and contract your ab muscles. Start rotating your body like a clock. Carry out 10 rotations on each side.

## Planks

Lie on the floor facing the downwards. Upper body should be supported on your forearms. Try lifting your entire body off the floor. Keep your toes in a straight line. Repeat twice and then break for 15s.

## Side work outs

Standing straight with your feet wide apart, approximately the width of your hips, slowly bend your knees while holding dumbbells in both hands. Lift your hands above your head and relax. Lean towards your right and raise your arms, hold position and then relax. Repeat for left side.

## Bicycle exercises

Lie on the floor and place your hands under your head and raise your knees off the floor. Bring right elbow towards the left knee while performing a cycling motion. Switch elbows and repeat

## Dumbbell bends

Hold a dumbbell in your right hand in such a way that your palm is facing the body. Feet should be at a shoulder width distance and slowly place your left hand on your hip. Bend upper body to the right side while facing the front. Bring your body back to normal posture and repeat with the left side.

## Perpendicular exercise

Lie on your back with your arms behind your back. Lift your legs over your hips at 90 degrees and breathe out. Then widen the gap between your legs. Breathe in as you lower your legs. Do a set of 5- 10 as you progress.

## Funky standing abs

Stand straight in the beginning. Next bend your knees and tighten your abs gradually. Push your pelvis forward so your back is curved. Return to original position and repeat the same by tilting your pelvis in the backward direction. Repeat the same in either direction for 15 times.

## Chair leg lifts

Sit straight with your back resting on the chair. Your back should be flat against the chair. Place your hands on the seat of the chair and slowly raise your knees towards your chest and put them back. Breathe slowly while performing this. Do a set of two and repeat 15 times.

## Crunches

The basic crunches are also essential for any kind of ab workout routine. Lie flat on the ground with feet placed firmly on the ground and place your hand under your head. Lift just upper body and hold for about 3 seconds. Repeat a set of 15-20 and break. Step up the number of repeats as your progress. This is a complete exercise as it targets not only the mid-section area, but the upper abdomen, the lower abdomen and the oblique abdominal muscles as well.

The ultimate goal is to build muscles and concentrate on burning fat. What follows what doesn't matter. If you are able to reduce weight before you begin your muscle toning work outs it is equally beneficial as toning up your muscles before you start cutting down on body fat. All depends on how motivated you are towards your goal of achieving that perfectly toned body.

Besides the regular work out and diets, you must follow an active and healthy lifestyle. Full body exercises like running, skipping or swimming helps burn fat while elevating your heart rate. Nutritious intake is essential to control on the fat intake in the body. Understand the importance of good and bad fat. A balanced diet is essential for losing that belly fat. Also, drinking plenty of water and limiting salt intake will help fight off stress levels and reduce chances of putting on weight.

Please check out my book series "HOW TO GET ABS" and get in the best shape of your life:

http://www.amazon.com/dp/B00SSFWCPA

http://www.amazon.com/dp/B00QJJFS1C

http://www.amazon.com/dp/B00SX58DUI

Check out my other weight loss and Nutrition Books at:

http://www.amazon.com/dp/B00QH7DY4Y

http://www.amazon.com/dp/B00RVX3KY2

http://www.amazon.com/dp/B00QDHXN7Q

http://www.amazon.com/dp/B00PP8OZJ4

http://www.amazon.com/dp/B00PO0IQIO

You can get access my Free Weight Loss Video at www.achieveitforyou.com

# YOUR 7-DAY TUMMY WORKOUT

## THE CRUNCH

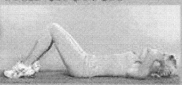 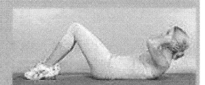

- LIE on your back with your knees bent, feet on the floor.
- PLACE your fingertips by your ears and keep your elbows pointing out to

the side, as you use your tummy muscles to 'crunch' and raise your shoulders off the floor.
- DO THREE sets of crunches.

## SIT-UPS

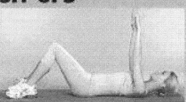 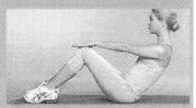

- LIE on your back with your knees bent, feet on the floor. Breathe in.
- AS YOU exhale, use your tummy muscles to bring your arms up and over at the same time as you slowly sit up.

- BRING your arms back and lower yourself to the start position, breathing in.
- DO TWO sets of eight repetitions, building up to three or four sets.

## CRISS-CROSS CRUNCH

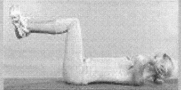 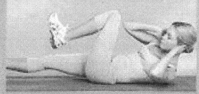

- LIE on your back as shown.
- AS YOU crunch (see the first exercise), bring your right elbow to your left knee and at the same time straighten your right leg without letting it touch the ground.

- BRING your right knee up to meet your left elbow and straighten your left leg. Keep up a continuous motion.
- REPEAT for two or three sets of eight.

## REVERSE CRUNCH

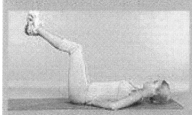 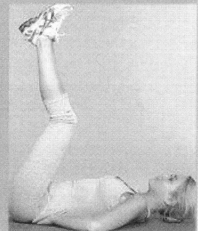

- GET in the starting position as shown, with your knees pointing up. Lower legs as shown above. Put your hands under your hips for support.
- USE your tummy muscles to pull your legs towards you and upwards (right). It's a small, subtle movement — you'll know it's working if you can feel your tummy tightening.
- REPEAT for two or three sets of eight.

How to lose fat?

The way to get lean and thin isn't through crash dieting or starving yourself for days. It is more about making the smart moves that help accelerate your calorie burn. Getting the technicalities right is very essential, we need to understand that harmful fat just doesn't mean a rounded belly or a wide waistline. Thin people can also show harmful amount of fat in their body. What we should be looking out for is the visceral fat. Most of this fat surrounds our different internal organs and a high content of this fat may spell trouble.

## Why is fat harmful?

A big part of understanding this problem is to get your diet right, not diet less. In fact experts suggest that the food intake should be in good amount and needs to be taken at the right hour and at the right interval. The ultimate aim is to fill your appetite with nutritious items and push out the empty calories, leaving you with a satisfied stomach and a healthy life style. If you add too many restriction to your food intake, it will end up lowering your metabolism to hold on to your existing energy. Unnecessary dieting may also lead to harmful effects like burning out your muscle tissues. This again results in slow metabolism killing all your hopes of reducing the body fat.

## What you eat matters

Focusing on your intake as mentioned above is a very important step in your endeavour to reduce. Your body needs a balanced diet of all nutrients, which include a healthy amount of protein. Protein helps build lean muscles. In a study done recently it was found, a daily intake of 0.5 to 1 gram per pound of your body weight is required along with regular work out to achieve that envious figure ultimately. Hence adding lean meat, yogurt, and some nuts to your regular meals will do you a world of good. The same research goes on to say that protein can act as a catalyst to your calorie burn rate, after every meal. It can up the rate by almost 30-35%.

## Go organic

Moving towards organic produce is another great stride in the direction of shedding that extra fat. Normal produce comes with artificial chemical and fertilizers aiding their ripening process. These chemicals interfere with the process of burning those extra calories. Or you can say fertilizers and insecticides will slow the process of losing fat. Hence, choosing organic food when it comes to your cereals, fruits, berries and veggies like potatoes can definitely help. These tend to use up maximum amount of insecticides.

## Fibre is the way to go

Incorporating a lot of fibrous food can be beneficial also. Fiber revs up your calorie burn by as much as 25%. This is a long term method and the results only show in case post regular intake. About 25 grams of fibre rich content should do the trick that means almost 3-4 servings of fruits and leafy vegetables daily.

Iron rich food is another easy way to keep away from putting on extra kilos. Iron is responsible for carrying the oxygen needed by your muscles to burn fat. You need to keep replenishing your iron stock to keep up the optimum metabolism level. A regular intake of Vitamin D is critical. Fishes, milk and eggs are rich source of Vitamin D. Ensure these are included in your diet. It will help preserve your muscle tissues.

## Other ideas that can help

Some research has also shown that lacking calcium can lead to slow metabolism too. Low calcium is a common problem in women so they should looks out for such signs. Regular consumption of calcium will keep up the metabolism level and aid in increasing the fat burn rate. Besides milk, specific fruits like water melon can also help burn extra calories off. The amino acid arginine is found in abundance in watermelons. This component helps in oxidation of fat.

Consuming red chillies have also been found to be effective in losing extra kilos. Chilies are supposed contain something called capsaicin which gives a kick to your metabolism. In fact a tablespoon of chopped chilies will up the metabolism rate by about 20%. So keep the chillies handy next time you make a sauce or any gravy.

## Drink Tea and Coffee regularly

Tea or coffee is another alternative when trying to burn extra calories. Caffeine the chief component in such beverages is a well-known stimulant for the nervous system and can push your metabolism up by 5-8 percent. Japanese research says the antioxidant catechins in tea provides the necessary boost.

## Give your lifestyle a boost of health

A lot of the problem is related to our overall lifestyle. For instance our sleeping habits. Studies between siblings have shown that the one who slept less had more amount of visceral fat content in the body. Stress levels can also add to your worries. Not sleeping well combined with high stress ultimately leads a tendency to put on weight.

## Be Active

Another major change can come from your activity level the whole day. If you are inactive more than 4 hours in a day (waking hours), it leads to shut down of the specialized enzyme that controls your metabolism level. So, it helps that you keep moving every few hours. Even a simple activity of getting up from your seat to get a drink from the cooler while at work will prove beneficial.

## Drink up

A very simple and cost effective way to keep the fat in check is by drinking lots of water. Drinking up to 7 glasses of water everyday can lead to losing about 50 calories. Drinking cold water is additionally helpful as the body puts effort into heating the water to match it with the body temperature.

## Common mistake that is to be avoided

A very common mistake we all make while trying to knock off those extra pounds is avoid eating our meals properly. We end up delaying them or skipping them altogether. While most of us feel comfortable with the idea of avoiding food and unnecessary weight gain, we forget that regular meals actually help us in the long run. Studies have proved that those who skip meals 4 times more likely to be fat. We also tend to forget about the most important meal of the day, the Breakfast. There is an old anecdote which says we should eat breakfast like a king and supper like a pauper. This holds true even in present times and should be adhered to strictly.

## Rid yourself of that belly fat

Washboard abs is what everyone desires for. Belly fat is extremely infamous for ruining that particular look you want to certainly get rid of that extra layer of tire. What is worse is this fat – also called the visceral fat- may settle on your inner organs and prove harmful to your health. So it's just not the looks but the health also which is at stake here.

**Start with some very effective exercises to get those dream abs**

**Begin with basics- The Crunches**

A toned and flat ab is out of reach for many but some regular exercises can help you reach your goal. The first that comes to everyone's mind are crunches. Regular crunches can be quite effective but the goal is long term and results may take a long time to surface. Sometimes crunching may not be the most effective workout. Crunches only affect the muscles on front and the sides of your abdomen, but it's still important to target all the muscles around the abdomen. This will give you perfect abs and benefit your thighs and lower back muscles also.

To uncover those amazingly flat abs and reduce your belly fat there are a series of other exercises, beside just crunches that can be done to produce wonderful and effective results. These are a set of three stabilization exercises which will create magic and show instant results. These exercises target the core area muscles, stabilizing the spine and pelvis. This gives you a better posture and removes pain in the back. These exercises ultimately burn more calories than your normal crunches and hence more effective over a period of time. See the great options below-

The first is the **side plank move**- Lie on your left side with your elbow under your shoulder and legs stacked. Place your right hand on your hips and try to prop yourself up. Maintain the position for 30-45 seconds at a stretch.

**Walkout from push up**- Get into the push up position with hands two inches wider than your shoulders. Maintaining this position walk to front and back. Do this 10-12 times to see great results.

**Alligator drag**- Get into push up position and drag yourself forward and backward. Rest for 60 seconds and repeat for best results.

It's important to complement the effort above with some other check list below. Please go through pointer listed below-

**Active Lifestyle is important**

An active lifestyle is the solution to belly fat problems. Hard core aerobics along with a regular hobby like cycling or swimming definitely works magic. A fun way would be to learn a dance form or go biking with your loved one.

## Yoga may be the solution

Yoga is another great way to relax and lose that belly fat. You don't need to be an expert in all the poses to be able to benefit from yoga sessions. Even simple breathing exercises can be very helpful. Easy breathing is the key to lowering the stress hormone – cortisol- level. Cortisol has been directly linked to belly fat.

## Meat – the storehouse of protein

Next time someone says go easy on the meat, ask him to stop feeding you with bad diet advice. Protein is essential and will go a long path in helping to rid those undesirable belly fat. Clinical research says as you age your body produces more insulin and insulin promotes storage of fat. A diet which is rich in protein content may protect you against the insulin resistance.

## Good fat or Bad fat?

Once you decide to bid adieu to belly fat, you need to start understanding your fat intake. Get this clear that not all fat is bad. Fat is good and essential for a balanced diet. You need to separate the saturated fat from polyunsaturated ones and consume accordingly. Polyunsaturated fat comes in the form of nuts, fish and different kind of seeds.

## Vinegar spells magic

A magic ingredient that has proven to be profitable is vinegar. Studies claim people who consumed a tablespoon of vinegar daily for about 2 months at a stretch showed drastic reduction in body fat. Drinking green tea is also hugely beneficial. Not only does it help reduce the body fat but acts as a cleansing agent for your body as well.

## Vitamin C has benefits too

Consumption of vitamin C is essential also in this attempt to lose that excess belly fat.  This vitamin helps balance out the stress hormone- cortisol. Vitamin C is also responsible for creating carnitine. This compound is used by the body to turn fat into energy. So make Vitamin C your fat fighting friend by consuming a healthy amount of oranges, kiwi and bell peppers.

## Breathe you way to health

Focus on your breathing during moments of stress or tension. Whenever you feel tired or worked up, check on your breathing pace. Most people take short and frequent breaths or very shallow slow paced breaths when tensed. Try and be conscious in moments of stress and control the speed of your breathing. Slow down the exhalation rather than focussing on inhalation. This will go a long way in reducing those extra few kilos off your belly fat.

## Cut down carbs

Cutting down on carbs in your diet is again a sure shot method of addressing the issue at hand. Studies have shown that a low carb diet lead to twice the weight loss compared to just low fat diets. Low carb diets also lead to reduction in water weight which ensure better and quick results.

## Other tips that can help

Some other small tips that help fight the bulge can be reading the label every time you buy a carton of juice or a soda. Try looking for the hidden calories and the sugar content whenever buying packaged food. Keep your lifestyle active, try to stand whenever the opportunity arises. Take calls while standing, get up from your workstation and go to the cooler to get your water. Start taking the stairs, mowing the lawn or any other activity around the house or in an office. One crazy idea would be to work out blind. With eyes closed, core muscles will have to add more effort to burn that extra calorie. Snacking on fruits and low calorie baked items also aids the process of burning that extra belly fat. Fun motivators like movies which inspire you to work out like- Chariots of Fire or Rocky- can also be a good idea. Start taking smaller helpings of food, use smaller dinner plates. Avoid insulin stimulator like potatoes at all cost.

## Great Abdominal exercises

Abdominal area covers the many interconnected muscles on our back, stretching down to your back, including our inner and front thighs. If you follow some of these simple to very complex work outs, you can be guaranteed to flaunting your washboard abs very soon

## Stretching and twisting-

The movement should be from your waist up. Whenever you twist, you must try feel a tightening feeling from one hip bone to next up. Always exhale deeply while working out. You must exhale thoroughly with every single breath.

## Two in one abs plus oblique work out-

Sit in a position where your thighs and torso make a V shaped structure. Lower legs should be crossed and lifted in the air. Take a dumbbell of about 5 pounds, hold it between your hands and swivel from the left hand to right, while maintain the V shaped posture. Do a set of 15 each and then repeat.

## Opposite arm leg reach out-

This work out can be done anywhere. Lie on your back with your left knee bent and right leg pointing towards the ceiling. Reach out to the ceiling with your left arm while keeping the right arm firmly by your side. Another kind of work out while maintaining the same position is worth trying. Don't move your shoulder or hips. Raise your right leg upwards and stretch the opposite arm to your left. Focus on your abs while doing so. Repeat with the opposite sides.

## Low belly leg reach

This particular exercise targets the torso area. Not to mention that a regular work out of this technique will lead to an enviable six packed abs. Lie down while facing up with knees bent at 90 degrees. Place your hands under your head and push towards yours knees. The knees should be stacked over your hips while you are doing your crunches. Break and Inhale for 5 seconds and then repeat. You can also extend legs and hold them together at 45 degrees. Hold this position for 45 seconds while trying to squeeze your lower abdomen.

## Teaser

An improvement on our last exercise. Lie on your back and lift your knees to 90 degrees with feet lifted. Tighten your abs when you inhale and raise your arms up and over your head. While exhaling, move your arms forward and straighten your body to form a V shaped structure.  Roll down then, bending knees and bringing your arms over your head.

## Donkey kickbacks

A killer work out technique that will prove to be supremely efficient. Kneel on your all fours with toes pointing inwards keeping back normal. Suck belly in towards your spine as you try to contract your abs and lift your knees a little above ground.

While keeping the abs engaged bring the right knee close to your nose and then kick out behind you. You should keep lower abdomens contracted and your hips should be facing the ground.

## Advanced crunches

Lie on your back while bending your knees. Place a small 3 pound dumbbell between your feet while tucking in your hands beneath your seat.

Focus on your lower abdominal area, trying to bring your knees inwards while raising your hips and shoulders slightly.

## The belly blaster

Lie on your back facing the ceiling upwards, with your knees bent inwards. Hold a dumbbell of maybe about 3 pounds between both hands. Keeping your right knee bent, stretch your left leg forward and move the dumbbell to the outside of the right knee. This will be like a part crunch and part twist position. Then pull in your left leg to meet your right leg and hold out the dumbbell towards the ceiling. Make sure your head and shoulder is elevated off the floor. Repeat the entire process.

## Oblique crunch

Lie facing downwards on a stability ball. Keep your feet hip distance apart and knees should be bent at 90 degrees. Place the right arm under your head and left arm on the floor to hold posture. Focus on your core and raise your left leg and try extending it. Next holding the same position crunch towards your bent knees, moving your right shoulder towards your left knee, stretching right leg forward at the same time. Repeat from top and switch sides after 15 reps.

## Scale pose

Sit in a cross legged posture with your hands placed next to you. Make sure you are comfortable. Your hands should be placed next to your hips. Then tighten your pelvic region, push in your arms and try to lift your entire body off the floor. Hold and count to 3. Then lower down your body back on the floor. This is pretty challenging but at the same time very efficient for the core muscles. If you can't lift your entire body, try taking support by placing your feet on the floor and lifting yourself up.

## Boat Pose

A very popular work out technique. Sit on the floor with knees bent and hands under your knees for support. Keep your shoulders pulled back and raise your legs till parallel to the floor. Knees should be bent all this time. You are now trying to balance on your seat bones. Try straighten your legs further and stretch your arms forward. Do this till the point you feel comfortable. Hold the position for about 15 breaths and then release the posture.

## Cross Leg crunch

Lie on your back with your legs straight on the floor. Keeping your torso steady, lift your hips and move them to your right. Lower your legs and repeat. Now bend your left knee and cross it on top of your right leg. Place your left foot on the floor outside the right knee. This will lead to a crunched up position and make the technique more effective.

## Tone it V hold

This exercises the twitch muscle fibres in particular. Sit while bending your knees. Grab on to the underside of your thighs with both arms. Lean back a little and lift your legs until parallel to the floor. Let go off the hands and try to maintain the posture. Try reaching your toes and hold for 8 breaths.

Please check out my book series "HOW TO GET ABS" and get in the best shape of your life:

http://www.amazon.com/dp/B00SSFWCPA

http://www.amazon.com/dp/B00QJJFS1C

http://www.amazon.com/dp/B00SX58DUI

Check out my other weight loss and Nutrition Books at:

http://www.amazon.com/dp/B00QH7DY4Y

http://www.amazon.com/dp/B00RVX3KY2

http://www.amazon.com/dp/B00QDHXN7Q

http://www.amazon.com/dp/B00PP8OZJ4

http://www.amazon.com/dp/B00PO0IQIO


You can get access my Free Weight Loss Video at www.achieveitforyou.com

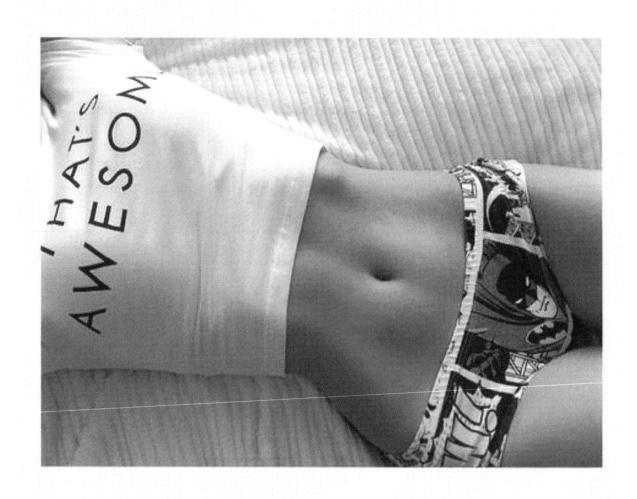

Ab exercises for men and women

While working towards your goal of perfect abs, we must keep certain fundamentals in mind. The best core exercises for men and women need to be diverse to make them most effective. Both genders approach core exercises in different manners.

## Different motivators for different gender

Research has shown women and men look at exercises with different goals in mind. Women look at work out routines with a holistic approach, with work out techniques like yoga usually involved in them. For men, exercise videos which involve pumping dumbbells, cardio work outs and building muscles will do the trick. Men love training with weights and benefit from some hard core work out techniques.

## Learn from each other

It's important that both men and women learn from each other's preferred techniques to get the best out of them. Both must involve cardio exercises to help reduce fat, or the muscles will never show. These cardio work outs are mainly strength training to help you build a better frame. It's essential that you don't keep working on the same techniques. Looking for variety while working out will keep you focussed and interested in your goals. Variety of ab work outs with different intensities should be your target.

## What to know when working toward great abs?

Keep the below pointers in mind while working out and you should be well on your path to a lean and hard midriff-

Focus on both lower and upper ab muscles while working out

Intensive work out is essential for fast results

Make sure that you feel the overall benefit. If your body doesn't feel right then you are doing it wrong

Reduce body fat, start burning those extra calories

Keep the tempo high and motivation up

Consistent work out and diet is necessary. Dropping out after a few weeks can't be an option.

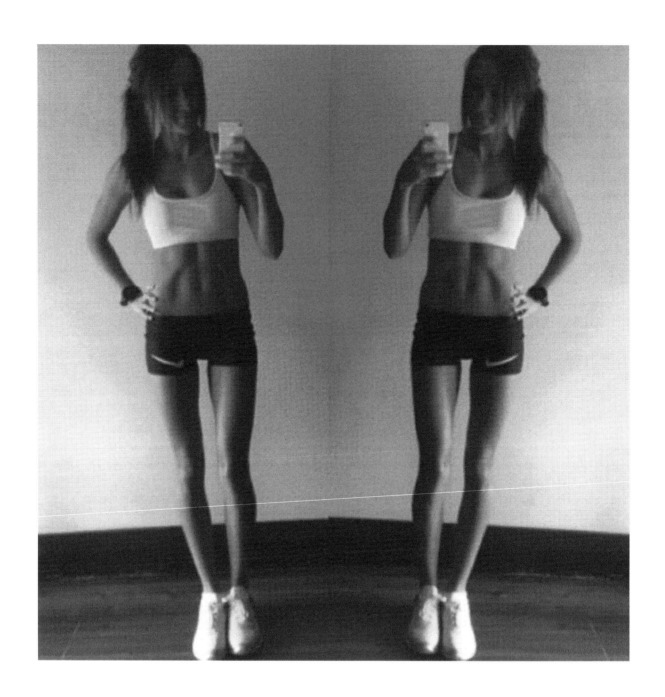

The magical Ab machines

There is no such thing as the perfect ab machine. Let's have this clear at the outset that perfectly flat abs can't be achieved through just work outs. It has to be combination of cardio exercises, the right diet and abs training. This will tone your core muscles and bring you closer to your dream of a desirable washboard abs.

However there are some basic work out machines which will definitely help you move closer to your dream of a desirable ab-

### Adjustable sit up machines-

This is the most conventional common machine found in any gymnasium. Meant for mostly sit ups, the handle angle can be adjusted to up or reduce the angle of the board. This helps us play around with the resistance also. Apart from sit ups we can also do crunches, twists and leg lifting. The seat or the bench needs to be wide enough to avoid injuries or any kind of strain.

### Ab slide-

A very powerful tool for training ab muscles along with arms, shoulders and the back. The ab wheel helps us perform a great core work out by stimulating our muscles every time we roll in and out. It is perhaps the perfect machine to work your lower and upper abs both.

### Bar-

Pull up bar machines are amazing tools for body weight exercises, very beneficial for achieving washboard abs. There are all kind of work outs that we can try out with this machine to work our oblique and abdominal area. Knee lifts and hanging leg raise exercises are especially productive.

### Stability ball-

This is essentially an exercise ball so not meant for ab work outs specifically. However, the ball can be utilized to carry out various kind of ab exercises. As the ball needs to be monitored regularly, it helps train the ab muscles better.

### Abs stretcher-

A great device for both advanced and rookie trainer. The strap sit comfortably around you and provide you the best work out motion possible. It is famous for the providing the best stomach muscle work out without requiring any special athletic skill to understand the technique. You can also try out the chin up bar move, which provides for a full range motion.

### Ab roller-

This machine is similar to the rocker system and targets the ab muscle in particular while providing adequate support to the neck and back. This machine is designed to be flipped over and be used for doing push ups. A complete machine for rock solid abs.

### Hyper back extensions-

This machine allows you to work both side of your midsections to strengthen your core muscles and stretch your lower back. The machine is adjustable according to height and size. The design is sturdy and durable. You can secure your feet firmly on the rollers while rubber caps at the bottom secure the floor beneath.

### Push up performance-

This device is special designed for upper body work out. The machine provides a smooth rotation, leading less strain on the joint and better muscle work out. Tire material tread provides great stability and prevents any chances of slipping.

## Semi recumbent ab bench-

This machine focusses on adding strength to core and back. The traditional crunches will only help a few areas of your abdomen. But this machine helps you target a wider area which includes lower abs, thighs and upper abs too.

Please note that these machines need to be handled under professional supervision. Working out at a gym or maybe with a personal trainer would be ideal.

Getting the perfect abs is extremely hard. It might just seem like a gift from god to some. Celebrities can be often seen flaunting great abs along with 6 packs or an 8 pack look, making us wonder how they adopt such looks so quickly. Mere mortal like us have to strive for months together and make the magic happen. The truth of the matter is if we put all our focus and time into it then it becomes a task of not more than 30 days. However, to stay motivated all through 30 days can be a hard task. Taking it on in the form of a challenge is a good idea. So why not put on your gym gears and start with the challenge.

## Why the challenge?

This 30 days ab challenge will tone up and boost your legs, thighs, and core muscles and add to your overall body strength. The challenge has four different exercises which needs to be completed every day and the time devoted to each exercise keeps getting added every day. This helps build your core muscles gradually ensuring that you are able to complete the final day challenge with ease. You just need to follow the chart and do the repeats the exact number of times as shown there. You can also download a fitness app on your phone and track your progress on it. This will keep the tempo up and running.

Some quick benefits of a 30 day challenge which makes a lot of sense-

The exercises can be done any time and any place you want. They are simple and don't require a lot of space

There is variety in the movement which can be aced by anyone. You don't need to be an expert to perform these moves.

The exercises are long enough to create a habit out of them. This will ultimately help you see results.

They are at the same time not so long and tiring that you burn out.

## What to keep in mind while taking the challenge

Remember to attain that healthier and slimmer body you must supplement the challenge by taking care of certain things. This will add to your stamina and maximize your performance. Remember to do the following-

Drink 3 litters of water every day

Give up on fast food, junk food and sugar based products like sodas

Eat healthy and organic food

Add brown rice and unrefined sugar to your menu. Toss out the refined packets

Bring down the size of your helpings. Reduced intake over a period of time can work wonders.


Please check out my book series "HOW TO GET ABS" and get in the best shape of your life:

http://www.amazon.com/dp/B00SSFWCPA

http://www.amazon.com/dp/B00QJJFS1C

http://www.amazon.com/dp/B00SX58DUI

Check out my other weight loss and Nutrition Books at:

http://www.amazon.com/dp/B00QH7DY4Y

http://www.amazon.com/dp/B00RVX3KY2

http://www.amazon.com/dp/B00QDHXN7Q

http://www.amazon.com/dp/B00PP8OZJ4

http://www.amazon.com/dp/B00PO0IQIO

You can get access my Free Weight Loss Video at www.achieveitforyou.com

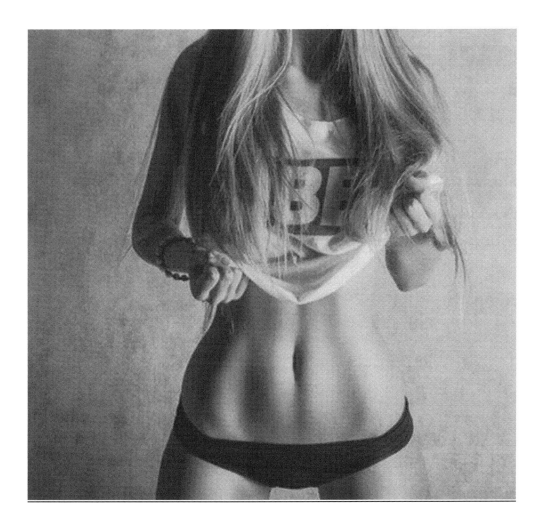

## Why 30 days may not be enough sometimes?

Please note that the intent behind this 30 day work out challenge is to strengthen your ab muscles in such a way that it's easily visible. Muscles definition varies based on body type and stamina. So the challenge cannot guarantee a perfectly sculpted body at the end of the 30 days but definitely get you closer to your dream physique. One should keep in mind that the challenge has to be combination of a great workout schedule and a proper balanced diet. The challenge needs to complete keeping your goal and endurance in mind. Pushing yourself too hard will demotivate you. Hence take the challenge wisely and complete it in as many days as you deem fit.

## An outline of the schedule has been represented below

Please see the schedule below. This will help you get started and bring you closer to the goal of that perfect ab

| Day 1 15 crunches+10 sec planks+5 leg raises+15 hip raises | Day 16 Rest today |
|---|---|
| Day 2 20 crunches+12 sec planks+5 leg raises+20 hip raises | Day 17 75 crunches+70 sec planks+50 leg raises+75 hip raises |
| Day 3 25 crunches+15 sec planks+10 leg raises+25 hip raises | Day 18 80 crunches+75 sec planks+55 leg raises+80 hip raises |
| Day 4 Rest today | Day 19 85 crunches+80 sec planks +60 leg raises+85 hip raises |

| | |
|---|---|
| Day 5<br>30 crunches+20 sec planks+10 leg raises+30 hip raises | Day 20<br>Rest today |
| Day 6<br>35 crunches+25 sec planks+ 15 leg raises+35 hip raises | Day 21<br>90 crunches+85 sec planks+65 leg raises+90 hip raises |
| Day 7<br>40 crunches+30 sec planks+15 leg raises+ 40 hip raises | Day 22<br>95 crunches+90 sec planks+70 leg raises+95 hip raises |
| Day 8<br>Rest today | Day 23<br>100 crunches+95 sec planks+75 leg raises+100 hip raises |
| Day 9<br>45 crunches+35 sec planks+20 leg raises+45 hip raises | Day 24<br>Rest today |
| Day 10<br>50 crunches+40 sec planks+25 leg raises+50 hip raises | Day 25<br>105 crunches+100 sec planks+80 leg raises+105 hip raises |
| Day 11<br>55 crunches+50 sec planks+30 leg raises+55 hip raises | Day 26<br>110 crunches+105 sec planks+ 85 leg raises+110 hip raises |
| Day 12<br>Rest today | Day 27<br>115 crunches+110 sec planks+90 leg raises+115 hip raises |
| Day 13<br>60 crunches+55 sec planks+35 leg raises+60 hip raises | Day 28<br>Rest today |
| Day 14<br>65 crunches+60 sec planks+40 leg raises+65 hip raises | Day 29<br>120 crunches+115 sec planks+ 95 leg raises+ 120 hip raises |
| Day 15<br>70 crunches+65 sec planks+45 leg raises+70 hip raises | Day 30<br>125 crunches+120 sec planks+ 100 leg raises+125 hip raises |

Please check out my book series "HOW TO GET ABS" and get in the best shape of your life:

http://www.amazon.com/dp/B00SSFWCPA

http://www.amazon.com/dp/B00QJJFS1C

http://www.amazon.com/dp/B00SX58DUI

Check out my other weight loss and Nutrition Books at:

http://www.amazon.com/dp/B00QH7DY4Y

http://www.amazon.com/dp/B00RVX3KY2

http://www.amazon.com/dp/B00QDHXN7Q

http://www.amazon.com/dp/B00PP8OZJ4

http://www.amazon.com/dp/B00PO0IQIO

You can get access my Free Weight Loss Video at www.achieveitforyou.com

Made in the USA
Middletown, DE
10 April 2021